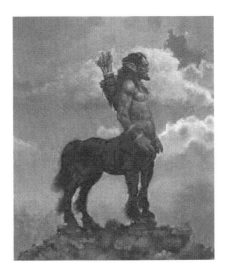

Hybrid LTC

Hybrid Long- term care Insurance-Making the Case

1. Long-term care insurance
   A. The need- high odds
   B. Stand-alone LTC insurance
   C. The expense-the numbers, demographics
   D. Tail risk-Retirement Smile

2. Planning Age-60

3. Hybrid LTC

Author's note

1. Long-term care insurance
    A. High odds

> There are many ways to consider your odds for needing long-term care. At age 65 the odds for an individual needing some form of LTC sometime are around 50%. If you consider the odds for one person in a couple needing some long-term care the odds increase

to at least 75%. That is why the thought of insuring for this risk make sense. The experience of having rates rise dramatically has soured the market for LTC insurance.

B. Stand-alone insurance

There are 3 main reasons given for stand-alone LTC insurance overpromising and underpricing.

1. Low interest rates -insurance companies assumed higher interest rates when they priced the policies. These low interest rates led to underpricing the policies.

2. Higher expenses- the costs of caring for the insured increased greater than the insurance companies assumed. Higher longevity and higher expenses led to underpricing the policies.

3. Lower lapse rates-the insurance companies assumed policyowners would lapse/drop their policies at a greater rate than they did. They assumed that 5% would cancel every year-leading to higher profits. They found that only

around 1% of policyowners lapsed their policies. This lower lapse rate led to underpricing the policies.

The experience of having rates rise dramatically has soured the market for LTC insurance.

(I do know someone who is keeping his "inexpensive" stand-alone LTC policy but is adding a hybrid LTC policy to supplement it.)

C. The expense-numbers and demographics
  1. The average LTC length of time for a female is 2.5 years.
  2. The average LTC length of time for a male is 1.5 years.
  3. 14% of LTC use exceeds 5 years.

4. For high income quintile, 22% of LTC usage exceeds 2 years.
5. 15% of LTC expense for 65 years old or older exceeds $250000.
6. The current 10,000 retirees turning 65 today are the future LTC recipients turning 85 in 2038!
7. By 2030 the over 65 population will exceed 20%.
8. The former unpaid caregivers-female non-workers -are now in the work force.
9. Families with no children or no children nearby will find it difficult to find unpaid caregivers.
10. LTC expenses are rising greater than inflation as demand is exceeding supply. (See 6-9 above).

Median Annual Cost of Long-Term Care

Adult Day Care	$17,680
Assisted Living	$43,539
Homemaker Services	$45,760
In-Home Health Aide	$46,332
Nursing Home (semi-private room)	$82,125
Nursing Home (private room)	$92,378

Source: Genworth 2016 Cost of Care Study

D. Tail risk-retirement smile

David Blanchett- retirement researcher at Morningstar- analyzed retiree spending trends. His data shows a consistent decline in spending from age 65-80 of about 1% a year as a retiree slows down physically and stops travelling as much. Around age 80- as a group- the spending starts to rise at a fast clip. This is the "retirement smile" graph.

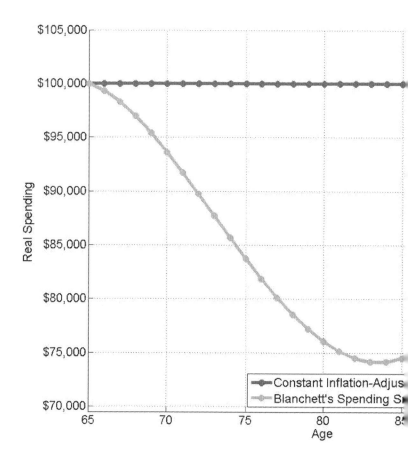

The chart above shows a constant decline in spending until it starts to rise dramatically in the 80's. This is primarily attributed to LTC spending. It is often referred to as health expense but most health expenses are covered by Medicare and Medigap. What this chart shows clearly is that if you have long- term care insurance -you can avoid the rise at the "retirement smile" in your 80's. Put another way, if your essential expenses are provided for the only major expense looming in retirement is long-term care. Addressing LTC lets you spend at a greater level from age 60-80 without having to worry about LTC expenses somewhere in the future.

2. Planning Age: 60

Ideally the earlier the better when buying LTC insurance but knowing when to buy helps to define the solution. In a perfect world age 50 would probably be chosen but there are so many other demands for the money such as college spending that I think setting age 60 as the date to focus on insuring for LTC insurance is a good compromise. The actual average age that people buy LTC insurance is age 59. (There are some products that allow you to fund LTC insurance from an IRA so starting after age 59.5 is helpful for that.)

If you have LTC insurance provided for at age 60, you can then dedicate time to understand Medicare/Medigap at age 65 and Social Security as late as age 70. Having 60/65/ and 70 as milestone age markers helps to simplify the retirement planning process which has so many variables.

Age 59/60 is the most popular age for new LTC insurance policies. For retirement planning there are only so many problems to focus on at a time. Until the children are self-sufficient taking care of their immediate needs takes precedence. Around this age is also when you might be taking care of your parents/relatives and understand the cost and importance of long-term care. Therefore age 60 -give or take 5 years- is a good sweet spot to solve this insurance problem. Since age 65 is when you will be dealing with Medicare/Medigap insurance decisions if you can get the LTC insurance squared away now you can later switch your focus to Medicare-which does NOT cover LTC!

3. Hybrid LTC insurance

   A. Guaranteed Premiums

   The major distinction between stand-alone LTC insurance and the hybrid policies is the premium guarantee. Stand-alone policies were underpriced and premiums have had a long history of increases. Many experts and actuaries say that the policies are priced correctly now but the premiums are NOT guaranteed and with potentially three decades of paying premiums and waiting to use the policy I do not want to take that chance. The design of the hybrid policies is different- they are designed as high-deductible policies and they have NOT increased premium prices in their history. Were they to raise prices, I suspect policies would stop being bought. Granted the guarantee is only as strong as the companies writing the policies so it is incumbent that the companies writing the policies are financially strong. I will write about financial strength and the high deductible design in subsequent chapters.

B. High deductible policies

Hybrid policies "work" because they are essentially high deductible insurance policies. You are essentially self-funding the first year or so of LTC expenses with your own assets. For those who can "afford" to set aside a sum of money that can be dedicated to LTC this "solves" the unknown future expense problem. Like all insurance policies the higher the deduction, the lower the cost to the insurance company.

Th chief criticism of these policies is that they are only affordable for the wealthy. In that case the only policies available are the stand-alone policies. BUT if you can afford to set aside a lump sum these policies not only are guaranteed but can be considered an asset on your balance sheet. Having these policies both addresses LTC in advance and can be helpful for estate planning by limiting an expense of unknown duration.

C. Lump sum amounts

To be able to buy a hybrid LTC policy it is best if it is paid for in a lump sum. Many retirees are unable to afford a high enough benefit level with a hybrid. If a retiree can afford a $50000 - $100000 lump sum from retirement assets without being a major strain on income, they should inquire about hybrid LTC. (Annual payments are possible if a lump sum is not feasible-but at rates higher than stand-alone insurance.)

Can you afford $50000-$100000? If this is only 3%-5% of retirement assets it should not be too great a strain on your retirement income. For this reason while hybrids are a great solution for LTC insurance, the vast majority of retirees cannot afford them.

D. Joint Coverage and Lifetime Benefit

There are policies designed to protect a couple so that the resources can be shared for LTC. Although the odds are 2-1 that the female needs greater coverage, many policies can add the male without doubling the cost. Whether using an annuity or a "second-to-die life insurance" policy, couples can share LTC coverage to cover both.

In addition to covering a couple, policies can be designed to pay out for the lifetime of the couple. Because the policies are designed as high-deductible, the insurance companies will design benefits that can cover the catastrophic events that might last much longer than the averages. There is an additional expense but this premium is guaranteed not to increase. Having a joint policy with lifetime benefits with premiums that don't increase is a great way to protect for the "tail-risk" of a much greater than average LTC event. Additionally, if this policy is in place the beneficiary will not delay in filing for benefits since there is no fear of exhausting benefits.

E. Growth of the hybrid policies

Stand-alone LTC policies have suffered from previous underpricing.

The early buyers-those most likely to do long term planning- bought policies and have seen their premiums rise. Even though many experts and actuaries think that the policies are now priced appropriately the reputational damage has been done. Hybrid LTC policies with guaranteed premiums have filled the void of the stand-alone LTC policies that can still raise premiums.

This graph from LIMRA shows the clear trend. The LTC market has evolved into a growing hybrid market replacing a declining stand-alone LTC marketplace.

The Rise of the Hybrids

As sales of traditional long-term-care insurance has declined, Americans are increasingly buying "hybrid" policies that add a life-insurance aspect to their coverage

Individual long-term care policies sold

■ Traditional ■ Hybrid

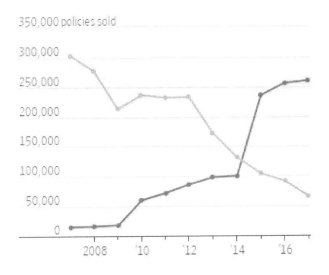

Source: Limra

Limra is the Life Insurance and Market Research Association.

Ownership of LTC insurance is skewed to the wealthy. 25% of those whose net worth exceeds $1 million have long-term care insurance policies versus 10% of the overall population over age 65. The insurance market with hybrid policies is definitely gearing sales to this demographic as an estate planning tool.

F. Refund-change mind

Many hybrid products which are designed as high-deductible policies allow a return of premium for the lump sum. This helps alleviate the fear if there is a change in the marketplace regarding long-term care policies as well as give the purchaser the ability to cancel the policy if their circumstances change or if they stop trusting the insurance company. Most policies have an additional premium to continue the benefits for a lifetime BUT those are not refundable. The lump sum can still be considered an asset on the balance sheet as opposed to an expense that can't be recovered. Combining a guaranteed premium with a return of principal is the marketplace's way to overcome the mistrust in the stand-alone LTC insurance marketplace.

G. Tax-free -HIPAA and Pension Protection Act

In 1996 HIPAA (Health Insurance Portability and Accounting Act) was passed. In addition to protecting patients' privacy it also changed how LTC was taxed. HIPAA expanded the definition of medical care to include "qualified long- term care service". This change made LTC insurance tax deductible by the employer and tax-free to the recipient-similar to health insurance.

Uniformity was brought to LTC insurance. To be classified as a tax-qualified plan, the insurance had to be guaranteed non-revocable and not duplicate Medicare.

In addition self-employed individuals could deduct their LTC insurance premiums.

To further promote private purchasing of LTC insurance Congress passed the Pension Protection Act of 2006 which enables individuals to exchange annuities or life insurance with gains into LTC policies and avoid taxation on their gains. This went into effect in 2010 and is only really beginning to be understood by the LTC market.

Expect Congress to continue to promote the ownership of LTC insurance through favorable taxation so that the government doesn't get stuck with the bill if Medicaid is the provider of last resort.

H. Funding of LTC hybrids-cash, IRA, annuities, Cash value

There are 2 hybrid LTC products- life insurance and annuities. There are quite a few ways to fund these 2 products.

1.Cash-either a lump sum or multi-pay-can be used to purchase a life insurance policy which is the vehicle used to pay for LTC expenses from the amount of the death benefit.

2. Cash -lump sum- can be used to buy an LTC annuity.

3. An existing non-qualified annuity can be exchanged for an LTC annuity.

4. An IRA can be used to fund a multi-pay life insurance policy which can pay LTC expenses.

5. A current life insurance policy with cash value can be exchanged for a hybrid policy-dependent on cash value and whether single or joint life.

The Pension Protection Act of 2006 made these conversions attractive with the favorable taxation bestowed on LTC insurance from 2010 going forward.

I. 5 sample cases

I chose 5 different hybrid cases. I used one single female and 4 couples of different ages to show some sample $ amounts possible from a lump sum. They are all whole life insurance that would provide a death benefit if not consumed by LTC expenses. I also added an annual "rider" that extends the benefit from 25 months to "lifetime". As these policies include purchasing life insurance there is some underwriting involved. These are sample cases that should not be taken as guarantees but as examples of what the cost of hybrid LTC insurance is today. This ebook's goal is to explain and demystify the hybrid LTC market so that potential purchasers don't get overwhelmed by the confusing terminology necessary to understand the product. If consumers are confused they will delay purchasing the product until it is too expensive or they are too unhealthy.

Case # 1

Age: 55

Single

Female

Non-smoker

Monthly LTC benefit: $4000

Lump sum premium: $65000

Annual "rider" (to make lifetime): $530

Death benefit: $133333

The lump sum of $65000 buys a death benefit of $133333. The monthly LTC benefit is $4000 and lasts for 33 months. With an annual premium of $530 the $4000 monthly LTC benefits last a lifetime. I didn't add an inflation increase as this $4000 monthly benefit is to supplement other income-not be the sole source of income for LTC benefits.

Case # 2

Ages: 55

Couple

Female and Male

Non-smokers

Monthly LTC benefit: $4000 (per person)

Lump sum premium: $56400

Annual "rider" (to make lifetime): $900

Second-to-die Death benefit: $133333

The lump sum of $56400 buys a second-to die death benefit of $133333. The monthly LTC benefit is $4000 and lasts for 33 months- either per person or whatever cumulates to $133333. With an annual premium of $900 the $4000 monthly LTC benefits last both lifetimes. I didn't add an inflation increase as this $4000 monthly benefit is to supplement other income-not be the sole source of income for LTC benefits. Compared to the first case this is a couple and is a second-to-die life insurance policy. (No death benefit paid until they both are deceased.) The LTC benefits cover both persons for a lower lump sum but a higher annual premium. The death benefit costs less because it won't be paid for a longer period of time-probably. This policy can cover a couple for a lower one-time price than for a single person!

Case # 3

Ages: 60

Couple

Female and Male

Non-smokers

Monthly LTC benefit: $4000 (per person)

Lump sum premium: $67300

Annual "rider" (to make lifetime): $1230

Second-to-die Death benefit: $133333

The lump sum of $67280 buys a second-to die death benefit of $133333. The monthly LTC benefit is $4000 and lasts for 33 months. With an annual premium of $1230 the $4000 monthly LTC benefits lasts both lifetimes. I didn't add an inflation increase as this $4000 monthly benefit is to supplement other income-not be the sole source of income for LTC benefits. Compared to the first case this is a couple and is a second-to-die life insurance policy. (No death benefit paid until they both are deceased.) The difference between this case and the second case is I raised the couple's age to 60 which increases the lump sum from $56400 to $67300 and also the annual premium from $900 to $1230. Once the annual premium is set however it won't increase.

Case # 4

Ages: 65

Couple

Female and Male

Non-smokers

Monthly LTC benefit: $4000 (per person)

Lump sum premium: $79700

Annual "rider" (to make lifetime): $1700

Second-to-die Death benefit: $133333

The lump sum of $79700 buys a second-to die death benefit of $133333. The monthly LTC benefit is $4000 and lasts for 33 months. With an annual premium of $1700 the $4000 monthly LTC benefits lasts both lifetimes. I didn't add an inflation increase as this $4000 monthly benefit is to supplement other income-not be the sole source of income for

LTC benefits. Compared to the first case this is a couple and is a second-to-die life insurance policy. (No death benefit paid until they both are deceased.) The difference between this case and the third case is I raised the couple's age to 65 which increases the lump sum from $67300 to $79700 and also the annual premium from $1230 to $1700. Once the annual premium is set however it won't increase.

Case # 5

Ages: 70

Couple

Female and Male

Non-smokers

Monthly LTC benefit: $4000 (per person)

Lump sum premium: $93500

Annual "rider" (to make lifetime): $2350

Second-to-die Death benefit: $133333

The lump sum of $93000 buys a second-to die death benefit of $133333. The monthly LTC benefit is $4000 and lasts for 33 months. With an annual premium of $2350 the $4000 monthly LTC benefits lasts both lifetimes. I didn't add an inflation increase as this $4000 monthly benefit is to supplement other income-not be the sole source of income for LTC benefits. Compared to the first case this is a couple and is a second-to-die life insurance policy. (No death benefit paid until they both are deceased.) The difference between this case and the fourth case is I raised the couple's age to 70 which increases the lump sum from $79700 to $93500 and also the annual premium from $1700 to $2350. Once the annual premium is set however it won't increase.

Waiting is not recommended as the health underwriting is harder to pass, the lump sum amount for the policy is higher and the annual premium to make it lifetime is greater. These basic formulas are useful to calculate if the cost of the policies are a good value for the protection you receive.

These are current examples in the marketplace and should not be construed as offers or guarantees. Instead of just talking theoretically about the cost of long- term care insurance I wanted to show real world examples to help explain hybrid LTC insurance.

J. The case for Hybrid LTC Insurance

If you believe that the cost of long-term care and the odds of needing long-term care are high it would be wise to insure against it by pooling with others so that a catastrophic expense would be muted. The stand-alone policies were underpriced and are now being replaced by the more popular but more expensive hybrid policies.

The stand-alone policies were affordable to the consumer but uneconomic for the insurers.

The negative aspects of stand-alone policies are positive aspects of hybrids. Hybrid policies have guaranteed stable premiums. Hybrid policies can be joint and lifetime policies. The lump sum for hybrids avoids the use-it or lose-it aspect of stand-alone policies and is refundable. Many insurance companies that wrote stand-alone policies are weak financially so it is vital that the hybrid insurance company is strong. (This can be discerned by looking at the Comdex (insurance rating) score. Hybrid policies can be funded in many ways-lump sum, IRA, cash value or ongoing premiums.

Hybrid policies' chief drawback is their limited appeal-not everyone can afford to part with a large lump sum. Unlike the stand-alone policies they are usually limited to those with sufficient financial assets unnecessary for retirement income. But for those who can afford them they are an excellent solution for long-term care expenses that can limit the unplanned expenses that can lead to the "retirement smile" later in retirement.

Author's note

It took me 3 years of researching
the product and the need for LTC

insurance to thoroughly convince myself that their guarantees were solid. The unattractiveness of even thinking about long-term care was offset by the elegant solution of a major retirement problem which makes planning for a prolonged retirement easier to achieve.

James McGlynn CFA, RICP ®
Next Quarter Century, LLC.

Email comments or thoughts to:

james@NextQuarterCentury.com

Made in the USA
Monee, IL
25 July 2020